MERCY MACHINE

a play by
Krista Komondor

For Dolores

CHARACTERS

MS. JENKINS, *early fifties.*
MORGAN FENSTER, *late twenties.*
VIOLET, *seventies to eighties.*
AGNES, *late sixties.*
MS.FOSTER, *fifties.*
BOBBY, *fifties.*
EMT, *forties.*
BRYCE, *forties.*
LPN, *thirties.*
SURGEON, *thirties.*
RALPH HAWKINS, *fifties.*
GUARD, *forties.*

PLACE

Mt. Sutton Center for Rehabilitation and Nursing in New York City.

TIME

The present.

MERCY MACHINE

Act I

ACT I
SCENE I

(Lights up on the office of MS. JENKINS, early 50s. She is preparing to leave for the day. She gathers ledgers, turns off her computer, and stuffs papers into a briefcase. A persistent knock is heard at the door.)

MS. JENKINS

What is it Millie?

(Knocking continues.)

Just give me a minute...

(Knocking continues.)

All right, all right, what is it?

(MS. JENKINS opens the door to find MORGAN FENSTER, late 20s.)

MORGAN

Ms. Jenkins--

MS. JENKINS

Yes. Who are you?

MORGAN

Morgan Fenster. I came about the Practitioner position.

MS. JENKINS

You're a little late.

MORGAN

I know, I just--

1

MS. JENKINS
I'm on my way out.

MORGAN
If I could--if I could have a couple minutes of your--

MS. JENKINS
I thought I'd seen everyone on the list. What time was our appointment?

(Silence.)

We did have an appointment.

MORGAN
(Hurriedly.) I called your secretary this afternoon--she said you were interviewing today and I came as quickly as I could.

MS. JENKINS
It's past 6.

MORGAN
I understand, but--

(Phone rings. MS. JENKINS answers.)

MS. JENKINS
Yes. *(Pause.)* Jimmy, I'm going to be a few more minutes.

(She hangs up the phone.)

MORGAN
I only want to tell you why I'm--why I'm the best candidate.

(Pause.)

2

MS. JENKINS
I'll give you three minutes.

MORGAN
Thank you Ms. Jenkins.

MS. JENKINS
Do you have a resume?

(MORGAN opens her briefcase, pulls out a copy of her resume and hands it to MS. JENKINS.)

Yes, yes...Fenster...I remember. Not much experience in long-term care.

(MS. JENKINS begins to hand the resume back to MORGAN. MORGAN does not accept it.)

MORGAN
I'm just starting out--but I'm a quick learner.

(Phone rings. MS. JENKINS answers.)

MS. JENKINS
Millie, yes. *(Pause.)* That's fine. It's ok.

(She hangs up the phone.)

(Mulling over the resume.) You're interested in full or part-time work?

MORGAN
I thought it was a full-time position.

3

MS. JENKINS
It's supposed to be but no one seems to want to take on the workload alone.

MORGAN
I'd actually prefer the full-time.

(Phone rings. MS. JENKINS answers.)

MS. JENKINS
Tricia, hi. I'm sorry but I'm on my way out. Give me a call around 9 tomorrow? Good.

(She hangs up the phone.)

So...you're not afraid to put in long hours?

MORGAN
No.

MS. JENKINS
We need someone who can spot declining residents before they get too serious. Are you comfortable with that?

MORGAN
I am.

MS. JENKINS
(Scanning MORGAN'S resume.) 4 months at Sullivan House. Why aren't you staying there?

MORGAN
Sullivan House is a temporary position. I'm looking for something full-time *(Pause.)* something permanent.

MS. JENKINS
Sullivan House has a vent unit, right?

4

(MORGAN nods.)

Do you have any experience working with the vents?

MORGAN
I helped manage their ten-bed unit.

MS. JENKINS
Then you're familiar with the difficulties that can arise.

MORGAN
I am.

MS. JENKINS
Good, good...Morgan, along that line...I need to
understand your philosophy.

MORGAN
My philosophy?

MS. JENKINS
Yes.

MORGAN
(Pause.) I want to protect these patients, to keep them
safe, and to...to help them live the best lives, the longest
lives they can.

MS. JENKINS
Good, good. At Mt. Sutton, we do that by offering the
best of both worlds--state of the art care in a home-like
environment. We have 5 vents now, and we're planning
on opening up another fifteen to twenty beds. *(Pause.)*
The reason I ask about your philosophy...you see, some
people--well, they just don't understand what we do
here, and I--I need to be sure that the clinician managing
the care of these patients is able to put herself in our

5

shoes--as well as the shoes of the family. We don't want any conflict, you see?

MORGAN
Yes, I see Ms. Jenkins.

(Phone rings. MS. JENKINS answers.)

MS. JENKINS
Ok, ok, I'll be right out.

(She hangs up the phone.)

I'm afraid we're out of time, Ms. Fenster.

(MS. JENKINS puts MORGAN'S resume into a folder with many other resumes and slips it into her bag.)

You'll hear from someone in the next few weeks.

(MS. JENKINS finishes gathering her papers. MORGAN stands.)

MORGAN
Ms. Jenkins, I'm willing and available to do weekend call.

MS. JENKINS
And you would do that for seventy thousand?

MORGAN
Yes, I would.

MS. JENKINS
(Smiling.) You're awfully agreeable.

MORGAN

I need to be here Ms. Jenkins.

*(MS. JENKINS picks up the phone and
pages the front desk.)*

MS. JENKINS

Millie, I'm going to have Ms. Fenster--

MORGAN

Morgan.

MS. JENKINS

Morgan. She's our new Practitioner. Get her paperwork
together for me and I'll have her fill it out right now.

(MS. JENKINS rises.)

All right Morgan, welcome aboard.

*(MS. JENKINS exits leaving MORGAN
alone on stage as lights fade to black.)*

ACT I
SCENE II

(6th floor of MT. SUTTON. We hear a voice in the dark.)

VIOLET
(Staccato and adamant, demanding. Not begging.) I want you to take me to my grandmother's house--take me to my grandmother's house. I want you to take me to my grandmother's house--I beg you, I beg. I want you to take me to my grandmother's house--take me to my grandmother's house. Please, please take--I beg you, I beg. I beg.

> *(Lights up on VIOLET, 70s-80s, sitting in a wheelchair. A pink bow wraps the gray hair on top of her head as one might generally associate with a Maltese.)*

I want you to take me to my grandmother's house. I want you to take me to my grandmother's house. I beg you. Please. My grandmother...she is so old, so sick, so alone. All alone. Please, please take me to my grandmother's house. I beg you. I beg.

> *(Lights fade out.)*

> *(Lights up on a private room. Standard hospital bed, standard cold fluorescent lighting. AGNES, late 60s, sits alone in a wheelchair.)*

VIOLET   AGNES

(Offstage.) I beg you, please take me to my

8

grandmother's house.

<table>
<tr>
<td>

(Screaming.) PLEASE, PLEASE, PLEASE! I beg you to take me. I beg. Please take me to my grandmother's house. I beg you to take me. I beg. PLEASE, PLEASE, PLEASE! I beg you. I beg! I beg!

</td>
<td>

(Yelling out the door.) Shut up you senile old bitch! Hey! Get me out of here--get me the hell out of here NOW! HEY!

</td>
</tr>
</table>

(AGNES throws the door to her room shut and quickly wheels herself into the center of the room.)

AGNES
(Muttering to herself.) This ain't no damned hotel.

(AGNES wheels herself over to the bed and pushes the red call button, pauses, then presses it repeatedly with a persistent forcefulness.)

MS. FOSTER
(Over an intercom.) What you want Agnes?

AGNES
(Screaming into the speaker.) Get me out of here!

(Long pause.)

Do you hear me?!

(Long pause.)

HEY!

9

(AGNES struggles with the wheelchair, attempting to get herself to a standing position.)

(Muttering to herself.) Said I was going to a hotel. This ain't no hotel. This is a damned nursing home.

(AGNES attempts to get herself out of the wheelchair. She crashes to the floor. MS. FOSTER, 50s, enters and quickly approaches AGNES to help her.)

MS. FOSTER
Oh mum, what you gone and do?

AGNES
(Virulently.) Get away from me!

(MS. FOSTER presses the call bell.)

MS. FOSTER
Bobby, Bobby, get in here. 625 cracked her behind tryin' to get out of the chair. Bobby, GET IN HERE THIS MINUTE! *(To AGNES.)* No sir, I am not breakin' my back pickin' you up.

(BOBBY, 50s, enters and scoops AGNES up into his arms.)

AGNES
No, not in the bed!

(He places her in the bed.)

MS. FOSTER
Listen, I've had enough of your screamin' Miss. You're stayin' with us now and that means you'd better mind

10

me rules. *(To BOBBY.)* Go call Fenster. Let her put up with this.

> *(BOBBY exits. MS. FOSTER examines*
> *AGNES for injury.)*

You'd better calm down. They fixed your left hip and now you go and fall on the right one.

> *(AGNES removes her shoe and throws it*
> *at MS. FOSTER.)*

Go ahead and be like that, see where it'll get you.

> *(MS. FOSTER slams the door and exits.*
> *AGNES pulls the cord on the light.*
> *Room goes dark. A thin beam of light is*
> *visible through the crack in the door.*
> *Loud conversation is heard in the*
> *hallway.)*

No, you can go in by yourself! The bitch threw her shoe at me--yellin' and screamin' and carryin' on.

> *(MORGAN enters.)*

MORGAN
Ms. Jones? Agnes? Can I come in? *(Pause.)* I'd like to talk with you.

AGNES
I'm through talking.

> *(MORGAN turns on the light.)*

MORGAN
You're upset.

AGNES

No shit. Who the hell are you?

MORGAN

I'm Morgan Fenster, I'm your Nurse Practitioner.

AGNES

You gonna tell me what the hell--this hole they put me in--who's responsible?

MORGAN

You didn't know you were coming here?

AGNES

You're a sharp one.

MORGAN

This is--they didn't tell you the truth.

AGNES

Damn straight they didn't tell me the truth. They told me "everything's gonna be fine. You're just gonna get a little exercise, a little rest. Get you healed up and back to your old self." Sounded like I was going to a damned spa. Leaving me off to die like--

MORGAN

You're not here to die Agnes. This is a rehabilitative center. You weren't sick enough to stay in the hospital and not well enough to go home. *(Calmly, encouraging.)* We've gotta get you stronger so you can get movin' and groovin' again.

AGNES

Hotel rehabilitative center my ass. This is a nursing home.

MORGAN
Listen Agnes, we have patients here who require all
levels of care. Yes, we have sicker patients who require
round the clock assistance, and yes, we have patients
who are nearing the end of their lives, but we also have
patients who are highly functional. Just like you.

AGNES
They gave you the same speech, huh?

MORGAN
What are you talking about?

AGNES
Must give the nurses and the patients the same speech.

(Silence.)

Cat got your tongue?

MORGAN
No. I mean, I--

AGNES
And what's with that ogre out there?

MORGAN
Ms. Foster can be a bit abrasive.

AGNES
A bit?

MORGAN
(Correcting herself.) The way she treated you was
uncalled for. We'll talk to her. You're a very
independent woman and I can only imagine how hard it
must be to have to rely on other people.

AGNES
You got that right. No way you can imagine.

MORGAN
Listen Agnes, we're putting you on a good program, and
I hear the food isn't all that bad. Just give us a chance,
ok?

(MS. FOSTER enters.)

AGNES
Hey Smiley, I want a cigarette, some bourbon, and get
me a phone!

MS. FOSTER
No drinkin', no smokin', and I hate to break it to you
missy, but the only phone here is a payphone--it's in the
hall. And don't ask me for no quarters neither because I
ain't got none.

(MS. FOSTER exits.)

MORGAN
Here, I think I can help you out...

*(MORGAN takes some change from her
pocket and hands it to AGNES.)*

AGNES
Thank you.

(Lights fade to black.)

ACT I
SCENE III

(The next day. Lights up on the nurse's station. VIOLET sleeps in a wheelchair against the wall. The phone at the desk rings. MS. FOSTER enters casually. She answers the phone on the fifth ring.)

MS. FOSTER

Mt. Sutton. *(Pause.)* Who am I? Who's this? *(Pause.)* Oh. Oh you want Mr. Ortez, do you? Well, he's not here. *(Pause.)* Well, I figure he'll be pushin' up daisies about now.

(MS. FOSTER hangs up the phone. MORGAN enters quickly.)

MORGAN

Ms. Foster.

(Silence.)

Hello?

(MS. FOSTER thumbs through a copy of The New York Post.)

MS. FOSTER

I can hear you. What you want?

MORGAN

I need to take a look at Mr. Lantz in 612.

MS. FOSTER

So take a look. I'm not stoppin' you.

15

MORGAN

I need your help.

MS. FOSTER

(Continuing to scan the paper.) Me? Whatcha need me
for?

MORGAN

I need help turning him.

MS. FOSTER

The nurse just did his dressing. You want me to turn that
fatty again? No no, I'm not going through all *that* again.
You'll have to wait 'til tomorrow.

(MORGAN stares at MS. FOSTER.)

I'm taking a little break. That ok with you?

*(MORGAN grabs a chart from the rack
behind the nurses station and begins to
leaf through its contents. MS. FOSTER
continues reading her paper.)*

MORGAN

How's Agnes?

MS. FOSTER

Must be doin' allright; she's downstairs givin' the
therapists a hard time--why don't ya go down there and
ask her?

MORGAN

Allright, I will. Goodnight Ms. Foster.

(Pause.)

What's wrong with Violet?

16

MS. FOSTER
Don't know. She ain't been fightin' me.

*(MORGAN examines VIOLET and
gently tries to wake her.)*

MORGAN
Did she eat her breakfast?

MS. FOSTER
Don't know. Feeders not in today.

MORGAN
She looks dehydrated.

*(MORGAN rubs VIOLET'S sternum
vigorously.)*

Hey, hello...hello Violet?

*(MORGAN checks VIOLET'S pulse. She
grabs the blood pressure cuff from the
desk and checks VIOLET'S pressure.)*

(With urgency.) I need to start an IV. Get me a setup kit.

*(MS. FOSTER goes to get the kit while
MORGAN continues to stimulate
VIOLET.)*

She should bounce right back once we get some fluids in
her.

*(MS. FOSTER tosses the kit onto
VIOLET'S lap and returns to reading
her newspaper.)*

Can you help me out here?

17

MS. FOSTER
Looks like you're doin' just fine.

> (MORGAN runs behind the desk to
> search for a bag of IV fluid. She is
> frustrated and struggles to locate the
> materials required to start the IV. MS.
> FOSTER puts down her paper.)

Whatcha need?

MORGAN
Bag of D5W.

> (MS. FOSTER digs into one of the
> drawers, hands MORGAN a bag of IV
> fluid and exits. MORGAN starts
> VIOLET'S IV and secures it. MS.
> FOSTER returns with an IV pole and
> hands MORGAN a small pillow to
> support VIOLET'S arm.)

Thanks. Let the nurse know I started this. I'll be back to
check her in a little while.

> (MORGAN exits. MS. FOSTER returns
> to reading her newspaper. VIOLET
> wakes up and begins to make soft
> grumbling noises. MS. FOSTER rises
> and wheels VIOLET back to her room.)

MS. FOSTER
Off we go Miss Violet, time for bed.

> (Lights fade to black.)

ACT I
SCENE IV

(The next morning. Lights up on a conference room. MS. JENKINS sits looking over paperwork. MORGAN enters hurriedly.)

MORGAN

I'm sorry I'm late. Things were a little crazy upstairs.

MS. JENKINS

Have a seat and let's get started. We have a lot to cover.

(MS. JENKINS consults her clipboard.)

We have 231 patients in house. 112-A, 210-B, 612-A and 515 are on bed hold; two admissions from Clarkson were canceled, 513-B was discharged to the community, and two patients were admitted to Clarkson. *(Pause.)* Morgan, what happened last night?

MORGAN

What do you mean?

MS. JENKINS

The patients you sent out.

MORGAN

Mrs. Pacheco in 801-A went out for respiratory distress-

MS. JENKINS

Again. Violet Watkins in 614-B was sent out. She was unresponsive?

MORGAN

She was dehydrated so I started an IV. We were keeping
an eye on her but she wasn't coming around so I sent her
out.

MS. JENKINS

Did she go out with the diagnosis of dehydration?

MORGAN

No.

MS. JENKINS

Thank god.

MORGAN

Why would it matter if she was sent out with--

MS. JENKINS

It would send up a red flag to the state and they'd be all
over us. *(Pause.)* So that puts us at…nine open beds.
Morgan, we need to watch our numbers.

MORGAN

Watch our numbers?

MS. JENKINS

We've got 9 out, and we can't have more than 12
vacancies.

MORGAN

Why is that?

MS. JENKINS

If we have more than 12 empty beds we won't be paid
for any of our hospitalized patients.

MORGAN

Why would we get paid if they're in the hospital?

20

MS. JENKINS
Let me break this down for you Morgan. See, if we have less than ninety-five percent occupancy we lose 'bed hold.' Do you know what that means?

MORGAN
No. What's bed hold?

MS. JENKINS
For every patient of ours that's in the hospital we receive three hundred and fifty dollars a day to hold their empty bed; seven hundred and fifty if they're on a vent. Bed hold can last up to fifteen days and it's good for three reasons: we need less staff; we don't lose any revenue; the patient can return to their original room--allowing for continuity of care. We're all right as long as we don't dip below ninety-five percent capacity. Do you follow?

MORGAN
Yes.

MS. JENKINS
Now, I'm not saying there's any reason not to transfer someone who really needs it. I'm just saying--seek my guidance first and we'll deal with these patients on a case-by-case basis. It's about achieving a balance, you see? *(Quickly.)* From now on I want you to alert me if anyone is at risk of being transferred out.

MORGAN
Of course. *(MORGAN looks at her watch.)* May I go now Ms. Jenkins?

MS. JENKINS
Not just yet. *(Flipping through her notes.)* We need to do something about our newest admits in *(Reading from a clipboard.)* 412, 322-B, and 625.

21

MORGAN

What's the problem?

MS. JENKINS

They're not participating in physical therapy.

MORGAN

(Consulting her census form.) The residents in 412 and 322-B have advanced dementia. They aren't able to follow commands, and--

MS. JENKINS

There's something you have to understand so that we can function here...see, these patients...they can't do a lot, but they can do a little.

MORGAN

A little?

MS. JENKINS

We only need to demonstrate that they can participate... a little bit for a little while. You're intelligent, you can understand that. *(Pause.)* All we need you to do is to certify that they continue to be candidates for therapy.

MORGAN

But--Ms. Jenkins--

MS. JENKINS

Morgan, with all the cutbacks at the state and federal level we're stretched as thin as it is. If you know of a better way to care for these people then my door is open, but if we fail another private home will take our place and then I'll be out of a job, and you'll be out of a job, and our people will have nowhere to go. *(Pause.)* Don't you see? That's just the way it is?

(Silence.)

MORGAN
Yes. I see.

MS. JENKINS
Good, good. So that explains two of them...what's going on with 625?

MORGAN
That's Agnes Jones. She can be a little difficult.

MS. JENKINS
Difficult?

MORGAN
She's had a rough time getting acclimated. I think she's depressed.

MS. JENKINS
Then we'll have to call in psych.

MORGAN
I don't know if that's really necessary.

MS. JENKINS
Listen, we're getting paid for these patients to get better, and that means they go to physical therapy. We need to do something because I'm not going to have the attorney general's office breathing down my neck again.

MORGAN
I think she could use a little one on one time. I'll ask the recreation staff to spend a little extra time with her.

MS. JENKINS
No no no--I'd prefer you take the lead on this; if she hasn't progressed by the time the surveyors pay a visit we want to make sure we can demonstrate that we've made an honest effort before calling in psych. See what

you can do; at the very least we need to document our efforts. Are we good?

> *(MORGAN nods in agreement. Lights fade to black.)*

ACT I
SCENE V

(Lights up on MS. FOSTER helping AGNES use her walker. She stands behind AGNES, holding her upright by a thick white belt fixed around AGNES'S waist.)

MS. FOSTER

All right mum...one two three, one two three.

(AGNES does not move.)

Ms. Agnes Jones...

AGNES

Don't rush me.

MS. FOSTER

(Calmly.) I ain't got all day...here, take hold of the handles.

(AGNES tightly grips the handles of the walker.)

Ok, now--

(AGNES takes one or two baby steps, then stops.)

C-mon mum... *(Joking.)* Hurry now so we can get you dancin' with your boyfriend out there.

AGNES

(Virulently.) Wait, wait...hold on a second!

MS. FOSTER

We gonna to do this or what? *(Pause.)* Let us go again.

AGNES

I have to go to the bathroom.

MS. FOSTER

Then you'd better start helpin' 'cause you can forget about me doin' all the work.

AGNES

I'm tired.

MS. FOSTER

And I'm tired of your excuses.

> *(AGNES takes another couple of baby steps, then stops.)*

AGNES

Wait a minute!

> *(MS. FOSTER looks up in frustration. They pause. AGNES takes a deep breath.)*

MS. FOSTER

(Slowly, with mounting impatience.) What's it going to be then? *(Pause.)* You ready?

AGNES

Uh huh.

> *(AGNES takes a small step forward. She struggles to hold herself up.)*

MS. FOSTER

Now get your legs--no no--hold yourself up.

26

(AGNES struggles to steady herself then gives up entirely, forcing MS. FOSTER to absorb all of her weight.)

Oh no you don't. You're dead weight and I'm not holdin' all of that up. I got enough of a job holdin' meself up.

(AGNES grunts.)

AGNES

(Exhausted.) I can't--

MS. FOSTER

(Fatigued.) Ms. Jones, you want to go to the bathroom or not?

AGNES

Just give me a minute…

(AGNES coughs and wheezes.)

MS. FOSTER

Listen mum, it's this way…the wheelchair is over there, we're over here, and the bathroom is within eyeshot. Which way's it gonna be?

(MS. FOSTER impatiently taps the leg of the walker. AGNES takes a short step forward.)

AGNES

Just hold--

(They stop.)

MS. FOSTER

You'd better start doin' some work. *(To herself.)* Won't do no therapy and I'm to pay for it.

> *(MS. FOSTER quickly sits AGNES onto the bed.)*

Here, you sit--take yourself a little break and I'll be back in a bit.

> *(BOBBY enters, drops a food tray on AGNES'S bedside tray table and exits.)*

There you go, eat your dinner sweetie.

AGNES

I'm not hungry.

MS. FOSTER

I'm not hearin' none of that. You gonna eat.

AGNES

(Pounding her fist on the table.) I don't--leave me alone. Get the hell out of here!

> *(MS. FOSTER stomps off/exits. In frustration, AGNES swings her arm back and violently sweeps her drinking glass and plastic water pitcher off of the bedside tray table. She picks up her food tray and repeatedly slams it against the table--she throws her entire body into this action. MORGAN enters.)*

MORGAN

Agnes!

> *(AGNES bangs her tray on the table.)*

28

Hey!

> *(AGNES bangs her tray on the table.)*

Stop it Agnes!

> *(AGNES bangs her tray on the table.)*

Agnes, cut it out!

> *(AGNES throws the tray across the room. A long pause. Quickly and detached, MORGAN picks up the tray.)*

You can't keep throwing tantrums Agnes.

> *(MORGAN places the tray on AGNES'S bedside tray table.)*

AGNES

Leave me alone!

> *(AGNES throws the tray across the room.)*

MORGAN

Fine.

> *(MORGAN turns to leave. AGNES begins to cry. MORGAN stops, her disposition changing. She takes a moment to refocuses herself. AGNES begins to cough/cry.)*

You've got to think about the other people on this unit. *(Pause.)* Agnes, are you ok?

AGNES
(Practically a groan.) Tired.

(AGNES coughs twice.)

I'm so tired.

*(AGNES falls backward onto the bed.
MORGAN pulls an oxygen tank over to
the bedside and offers the mask to
AGNES.)*

MORGAN
Here, take a couple of deep breaths.

*(AGNES puts the mask to her face and
breathes deeply.)*

AGNES
How much longer is this gonna go on?

MORGAN
When you're strong enough to use a walker you'll be
strong enough to go home.

AGNES
I can't.

MORGAN
I know it's slow, but--

(AGNES coughs and wheezes.)

AGNES
I'm so out of breath.

MORGAN
You'll breathe better if you're sitting up.

                        AGNES
Will you help me?

                        MORGAN
Of course I'll help you. *(Pause.)* All right, now we just
need to pull you up a little. I'll lift and you push, ok?

                        AGNES
I can't--

                        MORGAN
Sure you can. Here, get ready--on three, okay? One, two,
three.

                        (MORGAN tugs on AGNES'S sheet
                        while AGNES tries to scoot up in the
                        bed. They make very little progress.)

(A little out of breath.) Almost. Let's try again. One,
two, three.

                        (They repeat the same maneuver with
                        success.)

There you go.

                        (MORGAN goes to the foot of the bed
                        and turns the crank to raise the head of
                        the bed.)

                        AGNES
(In a hushed, ominous tone.) The nurse says I've got--
I've got sores on my back.

                        MORGAN
I know. She told me. *(Pause.)* Let's have a look, ok?

                          31

                              AGNES
I'd rather--

                              MORGAN
I promise it'll be quick.

                              (MORGAN goes over to the hand
                              sanitizing dispenser, presses the lever a
                              couple of times, and rubs her hands
                              vigorously. AGNES rolls over to face the
                              audience. MORGAN opens AGNES'S
                              gown in the back. We see a look of great
                              concern on MORGAN'S face.)

                              AGNES
How is it?

                              MORGAN
(Lying.) Fine. It's small, but--

                              AGNES
But?

                              MORGAN
(Pause.) I'm not too crazy about the way it looks.

                              (MORGAN covers the wound and moves
                              AGNES to a sitting position. She goes to
                              the sink and washes her hands.)

They need to turn you more often.

                              AGNES
Good luck. They come in here and it's in and out, in and
out; pop a head in and out they go.

                              MORGAN
(Motioning to the tray that lies against the wall.) I see

                                32

you're not very hungry.

                    AGNES
You try eating that shit.

            (*MORGAN takes note of the food.*)

                    MORGAN
I'll talk to dietary--or--is there someone we can call to
bring in a couple of your favorites?

                    AGNES
I'm no good to anyone anymore.

                    MORGAN
I saw your son's name on your chart but I couldn't find
his number. Do you have it?

                    AGNES
He doesn't have a phone.

                    MORGAN
Where does he live?

                    AGNES
Upstate.

                    MORGAN
Why haven't I seen him?

                    AGNES
He's busy lookin' for work.

                    MORGAN
What does he do?

                    AGNES
A little of this…a little of that...

(AGNES coughs and wheezes violently.)

I've got a picture of him over there--in my pocketbook.

> *(AGNES motions for MORGAN to get
> her purse out of the nightstand.
> MORGAN hands AGNES her purse, and
> AGNES rustles through the bag to find
> the photograph. She shows the photo to
> MORGAN.)*

MORGAN

He's very handsome.

AGNES

Takes after his father.

> *(MORGAN holds the photo up to
> AGNES.)*

MORGAN

I don't know...he resembles you quite a bit...the
mouth...and the eyes. You must love him very much.
(Pause.) When's the last time you saw him?

AGNES

He writes now and then.

MORGAN

We should probably finish your dressing.

AGNES

Your turn--you got any pictures of your sweetheart?

> *(MORGAN laughs quietly.)*

MORGAN

I don't have one.

34

                              AGNES
A pretty girl like you?

                              MORGAN
Nah.

                              AGNES
Why not?

                              MORGAN
Too much to do.

                              AGNES
Bullshit. What's there to do? *(Pause.)* This place?

                              MORGAN
People need me.

                              AGNES
Girl, you gotta get out of here and go find yourself a fine
piece of--

                              MORGAN
Agnes--

                              AGNES
It's all gonna dry up. You don't want to get no cobwebs
up there.

                              MORGAN
Please Agnes…

                              AGNES
Girl, are you crazy? You've just gotta go and jump on it!

                              *(AGNES makes an obscene gesture with
                              her hands.)*

                              35

MORGAN
(Embarrassed.) Agnes!

AGNES
I never heard of such a thing.

(AGNES coughs and wheezes violently.)

MORGAN
Agnes--hey, you okay?

AGNES
I--

*(MORGAN listens to AGNES'S lungs
with a stethoscope.)*

MORGAN
I'll order another treatment.

AGNES
(Recovering a bit.) Doesn't matter.

MORGAN
What?

AGNES
They won't give it to me.

MORGAN
I'll do it myself. Hold on, I'll get the nebulizer.

(MORGAN rises to exit.)

AGNES
I want water.

MORGAN

Here...

*(MORGAN pours a glass of water from
a pink plastic pitcher, places a straw in
the glass and lifts it up to AGNES'S
lips.)*

All right?

AGNES

Yeah, I--I think so.

(MORGAN gently rubs AGNES'S back.)

MORGAN

I'll give you a treatment and then we'll have another
listen.

AGNES

Why're you doin' all this for me?

MORGAN

It's my job.

AGNES

All this ain't your job. Why you bein' so nice to me?

MORGAN

My grandmother was in a place like this.

AGNES

Is she still?

(MORGAN shakes her head no.)

How long ago did she...

MORGAN

About 6 months, 6 months ago.

AGNES

I'm sorry.

(MORGAN looks at her watch.)

MORGAN

If we can catch the x-ray tech I'd like him to get a picture of your lungs.

AGNES

No. I don't want them botherin' me…don't need no one probin' me.

MORGAN

Agnes--

AGNES

NO WAY!

MORGAN

Agnes--

AGNES

What time is it?

MORGAN

7:00.

AGNES

Good. Time for you to get outta here, go!

MORGAN

I have to finish your--

AGNES

Bye!

MORGAN

Agnes--

AGNES

So long!

MORGAN

I need to finish your dressing.

AGNES

Please, no. *(With trepidation.)* It hurts.

MORGAN

I'll be gentle.

AGNES

Promise? *(Pause.)* All right. *(Preparing herself.)* Ok.

>*(MORGAN helps AGNES turn onto her side.)*

I feel like I'm…like I'm losing sense of myself…

>*(MORGAN cleanses the wound, covers it with gauze, and applies tape.)*

I don't know what's gonna happen to me…

MORGAN

What do you mean Agnes?

AGNES

This morning I was lookin' for my friend Francis 'cause I heard she'd come back from the hospital. We used to talk in the day room--hadn't seen her since she went off to the--off to the hospital. I asked the nurse up there on eight what room she was in and I went in to see her, and she--she was in there but it--no, it wasn't her--it looked nothin' like her, nothin' like Francis. Francis wasn't--it was NOT HER. That woman, the woman layin' in the bed, she didn't look alive no more…layin' in the bed, layin' there like a corpse and--and she had all these hoses comin' out of her, and the hoses…they were hooked up to this loud machine pumpin' away and she had all these tubes comin' out of her and I saw--she had her eyes open and I went over to see her, and--she--she looked at me and she scared the hell out of me the way she was lookin' at me. I got--I had to get--get myself outta there…all I could think was…what the hell happened to her, and why isn't anyone else there, and why doesn't someone try to HELP HER?

MORGAN
I'm so sorry Agnes. *(Pause.)* You see Agnes, sometimes people get really sick and…instead of passing on--well, people try to keep them alive.

AGNES
Why would anyone do that?

MORGAN
People can be so afraid to lose someone they love--they think if we'd all just try harder they won't have to lose them, and they think that putting a person on that type of machine…even though they may never get off of it…that it's better than having them die.

AGNES
I don't ever want to be like that.

MORGAN
(Contemplates this with difficulty.) Agnes, when you
were admitted did anyone talk to you about an advance
directive...a healthcare proxy or a living will?

AGNES
Proxy, living? I don't know, I mean, I think--when I
came here they were talkin' about how, how what if
something bad happened, but I just--you know, I don't
wanna jinx myself.

MORGAN
Do you know what having an advance directive means?
It gives you a choice. If you don't choose, someone else
will do it for you. It's like a plan Agnes.

AGNES
A plan?

MORGAN
We need to plan for what could happen. I'm not saying it
will happen, but--what I'm trying to say is--if...if your
heart stopped beating or you stopped breathing--there are
things that can be done to bring you back, things we can
do to keep you alive.

AGNES
Those machines...

MORGAN
Right. See, if you don't have a plan and you stop
breathing...one of those machines would breathe for
you.

AGNES
Would you want that?

MORGAN
I don't know what I'd want.

AGNES
Would you trust someone you don't know to decide for you?

MORGAN
I don't think I would.

AGNES
Well, I don't want none of that.

MORGAN
You wouldn't want to be resuscitated and you wouldn't want any artificial--

AGNES
Promise me I won't be kept on like that. Promise that'll never happen to me!

(Pause.)

MORGAN
Ok. I'll talk to the social worker and we'll get the paperwork in order, but we really need to get ahold of your son to make sure we're all in agreement. Do you have any idea how we can reach him?

AGNES
Like I said, he doesn't have a phone.

MORGAN
I know, but it's important that we find him.

AGNES
His address--I have to have it somewhere. I used to write to him, used to help him out.

MORGAN
Help him out?

AGNES
Used to give him my check before this place. This place
they take it all. It's expensive keepin' me alive.

MORGAN
Don't talk like that.

AGNES
How many people do you think have--have died in this
bed before me?

MORGAN
You don't need to think about that--

AGNES
(Laughing.) Like on that commercial about the roach
motel, huh? "Roaches go in but they don't come out?"
(Pause.) My father, he used to say "whenever I can't
wipe my own ass, just shoot me."

*(AGNES laughs sardonically, then
begins to cry/cough.)*

My god, what would he say about me now?

(Lights fade to black.)

*(Lights up on VIOLET seated in a
wheelchair in the hallway. Behind her is
wallpaper with pink flowers and green
stripes. A 'painting' of a sunrise is
screwed into the wall. VIOLET eats
cookies out of a box, making lip-
smacking sounds while savoring the
cookies. AGNES wheels herself into the
hallway. She looks significantly weaker
and coughs. The coughs are intermittent
at first. As the scene progresses, they
become quite violent.)*

AGNES
(Seeing Violet.) Oh my god.

(AGNES turns to exit.)

VIOLET
(Simply.) Do you want a cookie?

AGNES
(Uncertain if she should respond.) Well…

VIOLET
They're very delicious.

*(VIOLET finishes her cookie, generously
licks her fingers, and returns her hand
to the box. She grabs another cookie
from the box and holds it out to
AGNES.)*

AGNES
No, you go ahead. I don't have much of an appetite.

                          VIOLET
Ok.

                (VIOLET eats another cookie.)

                          AGNES
Thanks anyway. *(Pause.)* I'm surprised to hear you so
chatty.

                *(VIOLET continues to make lip-
                smacking sounds.)*

You always seem so upset.

                          VIOLET
Upset?

                          AGNES
You know, about your grandmother.

                          VIOLET
(Simply.) She has no one and she is all alone.

                          AGNES
Where does she live?

                          VIOLET
Up that little road. She has a house, a little cabin. I live
there with her.

                          AGNES
Is that so.

                          VIOLET
Um, yes…but I have to get home soon. Are you sure
you don't want a cookie?

                            45

                    AGNES
No, I'm all right.

                    VIOLET
Would you take me home?

                    AGNES
I don't know where home is anymore.

                    VIOLET
I have to get home.

                    AGNES
Yeah, I know--home to your grandmother's house.

                    VIOLET
(A little more demanding.) Please take me there.

                    AGNES
I can't.

                    VIOLET
(Escalating, strong, adamant.) Please. I beg you.

                    AGNES
I said I CAN'T.

                    VIOLET
You must help her--

                    AGNES
Listen, calm down, just--

                    VIOLET
I beg you, I BEG--

                    AGNES
Just shut up.

VIOLET

(Demanding.) Please. Please. You must take me to my grandmother's house!

AGNES

Not again.

VIOLET

I beg you, I beg!

AGNES

This is where I check out.

(AGNES attempts to wheel herself away but VIOLET grabs hold of her shawl. AGNES fights to free herself.)

HELP!

(VIOLET tightens her grasp on AGNES'S shawl making it even more difficult for AGNES to breathe.)

VIOLET

You must help her!

AGNES

Somebody please help me. Please!!!

VIOLET

She is sick, and old, and all alone.

(BOBBY enters.)

BOBBY

I'm not gonna take another eight hours of this shit.

47

VIOLET

You must take me; you must help her. PLEASE!

*(BOBBY grabs VIOLET and pries her
fingers off of AGNES'S shawl. AGNES
is released. BOBBY grabs the box of
cookies from VIOLET and taunts her
with a cookie.)*

BOBBY

Hey Violet, you want a cookie? You want a fucking
cookie?

VIOLET

Please take me!

*(MORGAN enters without being
noticed.)*

BOBBY

You want to know where your grandmother is Violet?
She's DEAD! Your grandmother's DEAD!

VIOLET

NO!

(VIOLET strikes BOBBY in the face.)

BOBBY

You stupid old bitch! *(Screaming offstage.)* FOSTER!
FOSTER, get out here and bring me a vest! Shit Foster,
call the shrink and let's get this bitch medicated!

(MS. FOSTER enters.)

MS. FOSTER

What's going on here?

48

                          BOBBY
Hurry! Get a vest.

> (*MS. FOSTER grabs a restraint vest
> from behind the nurses' station and
> throws the vest to BOBBY who begins to
> aggressively put it on VIOLET.*)

                          MORGAN
(To BOBBY.) Get away from her.

> (*MORGAN pushes BOBBY aside and
> removes VIOLET'S vest.*)

(To MS. FOSTER.) Please take Violet to her room.
Please try to calm her.

> (*MS. FOSTER exits with VIOLET.
> MORGAN turns to BOBBY. They look at
> each other for a moment. BOBBY exits.*)

Agnes. Agnes, it's ok. You're safe.

> (*AGNES coughs and sputters. She looks
> significantly weaker.*)

Agnes, are you ok?

                          AGNES
I'm fine.

> (*MORGAN puts the back of her hand on
> AGNES'S forehead.*)

                          MORGAN
You're burning up.

                            49

(AGNES continues to cough. MORGAN listens to AGNES'S chest with a stethoscope.)

Your lungs sound so much worse. Agnes, I'm going to transfer you to the hospital. It's going to be ok; they can give you stronger medicine than we can give you here.

(MS. FOSTER enters briskly, sees MORGAN, then turns to exit.)

Foster, stop!

(MS. FOSTER stops and slowly turns around to face MORGAN. AGNES feebly wheels herself offstage.)

MS. FOSTER
(Stoic.) Yes, Ms. White coat?

MORGAN
What do you think you're doing?

MS. FOSTER
Excuse me?

MORGAN
You can't treat people like this.

MS. FOSTER
Treat them? How'm I treatin' them?

MORGAN
Like animals.

MS. FOSTER
Whoa, now hold on.

MORGAN

I've suspected that this sort of thing had been going on
but I didn't want to believe it.

MS. FOSTER

I'm not sure I know what you're talkin' about.

MORGAN

Bobby provoked her.

MS. FOSTER

She's got the dementia--

MORGAN

Yes, she has dementia, but he had no right to--

MS. FOSTER

Did she hit Bobby?

MORGAN

That's irrelevant.

MS. FOSTER

I said 'did she hit him?'

MORGAN

Yes, but--

MS. FOSTER

But what?

MORGAN

Who am I talking to? I just said she has dementia--

MS. FOSTER

And I said I saw that old woman beatin' the hell out of
Bobby.

51

MORGAN

That makes it ok for him to do whatever he likes? What kind of person are you? You're hired to care for Violet, not to hurt her.

MS. FOSTER

Don't think you can stand back and be judgin' me 'cause you've got no idea.

MORGAN

Oh, I don't?

MS. FOSTER

You don't know what it's like to be in our shoes.

MORGAN

We work in the same facility with the same residents. There is one primary difference--I don't terrorize them.

MS. FOSTER

There's no way you can compare yourself to me. You listen to me missy...the life we have, the job we do, it's hard. When your day is done don't you go home, put your feet up, eat your Ben and Jerry's and shrug off the day? Maybe go out for a little drinkin' and dancin' with your girlfriends, and maybe even get a little nookie? *(Pause.)* Do you know what I do?

MORGAN

No, Ms. Foster, what do you do?

MS. FOSTER

I go to me next job. On my feet another eight hours and then home to try to give me family some care. What do you think of that missy?

MORGAN

That's your choice.

52

MS. FOSTER

I ain't got no choice Miss.

MORGAN

Everyone has a choice.

MS. FOSTER

Do they?

(MS. FOSTER circles MORGAN.)

Maybe--if they're lucky enough to come from a
privileged family--yes, in that case there certainly would
be a choice; no doubt about that.

(MORGAN is silent.)

(Slowly, strong.) Minimum wage. You know what that
means missy? Seven twenty-five an hour. They don't
pay me more because they don't have to, and if they
could pay me less you'd better believe they would.

MORGAN

If you wanted to--

MS. FOSTER

Seven twenty-five to wipe their asses, to clean their
vomit, to get attacked by some psycho? How much do
you get paid to write your little notes, to write your little
orders for us to bow down and carry out?

MORGAN

This is pointless. I'm getting Ms. Jenkins. You won't
have to worry about how hard you've got it anymore.

MS. FOSTER

You think she doesn't know what goes on here?

(Silence.)

MORGAN
What do you mean?

MS. FOSTER
She's gonna replace us? You really believe that? No no…she's got a good deal goin' on here. Bodies, she needs bodies, and ours are as good as any other.

MORGAN
Any of these residents could be your mother, your father--

MS. FOSTER
Not my mother. No sir, my mother she stays with me. I keep and I care for my own. Who else gonna care for your own flesh and blood? I don't give em' over to no one else and certainly not to a place like this. She's family. *(Pause.)* Not like them.

> *(MS. FOSTER motions to a rack of charts.)*

MORGAN
How's she different?

MS. FOSTER
Listen missy, I'm no big shot wearin' no fine pressed suit or a white coat for that matter. No, I'm just a woman tryin' to get by the best she can. And to me 605-A is no different from 615-B or Mr. 635 in his private room.

MORGAN
(Simply.) These are human beings.

54

MS. FOSTER

Where? I don't see no human beings. I see 'residents,' I
see 'inmates.' And that's all I see because *(Pause.)* if I
think they're anything else *(Pause.)* don't you think I'd
lose me mind?

> *(MS. FOSTER exits. MORGAN is left
> alone on stage. Lights fade to black.)*

ACT I
SCENE VII

(Lights up on the nurse's station. MS. JENKINS is on the phone pacing back and forth.)

MS. JENKINS
Well why can't you send the ambulance back? No. There's no emergency. It was a false alarm. No. There's no emergency. Just send it back!

(MORGAN enters. MS. JENKINS hangs up the phone.)

What's going on here?

MORGAN
What do you mean?

MS. JENKINS
Agnes--why wasn't I notified?

MORGAN
We have to get her out.

MS. JENKINS
Why?

MORGAN
What do you mean?

MS. JENKINS
We discussed this--you first contact me and I will decide if a resident needs to be hospitalized.

MORGAN
This is serious--I didn't think I needed to--

56

MS. JENKINS
That's the problem; you didn't think.

MORGAN
This isn't the time.

MS. JENKINS
This is not the way we do things around here.

(An EMERGENCY MEDICAL
TECHNICIAN, 40s, enters.)

EMT
Ok, what've we got here?

MORGAN
71-year-old female with a history of COPD. 104.1 temp
and a respiratory rate of 25; she became tachypnic half
an hour ago. PO Levaquin was started four days ago.
Initial response was good but today she developed a
productive cough with green sputum. We've been
suctioning her and giving her O2 but her sats are still
down.

EMT
What's she running?

MORGAN
60% on four liters O2.

EMT
She a DNR?

MORGAN
(Hesitant.) No.

EMT
Shit. (Pause.) Ok, let's hope for a smooth ride.

(The EMT walks briskly toward AGNES'S room.)

MORGAN

You still don't think she needs to go to the hospital?

MS. JENKINS

That's beside the point. Don't start thinking you're the one in charge here because you're not. Next time you talk to me.

(MS. JENKINS exits. Lights fade to black.)

Act II

ACT II
SCENE I

(Lights up on a conference room during morning report.)

MS. JENKINS
We've got 8 on bed hold and *(Consults her clipboard.)* 1, 2, 3, 4 empty beds. I'll call Clarkson and see how fast we can get...701 and 716-B. I'll see how soon can we get them back, but--it looks like 701's only on his eighth day. *(Pause.)* That woman--Jones, the one you sent out via 911, she's on her way back.

MORGAN
How can Agnes come back so soon?

MS. JENKINS
She's stable.

MORGAN
But her breathing--

MS. JENKINS
Is no longer an issue; she's on a vent now.

(Lights up stage right. AGNES'S bed is wheeled in by BOBBY. MS. FOSTER follows with the ventilator.)

Standard setup--she's got a peg tube in place so we won't have to worry about replacing an NG...and it looks like she's coming back with a Stage IV ulcer.

MORGAN
When she left here it was a Stage II. In two weeks she went from a Stage II to a Stage IV?

59

MS. JENKINS
If it needs debrided we can get one of their surgeons to drop by.

MORGAN
If it needs debrided--wouldn't they have done that while she was at Clarkson?

(Silence.)

MS. JENKINS
Things like that can easily be done in our facility. *(Pause.)* Just go up and do what you need to do; remember to take pictures and measurements so we can document that it didn't happen here.

MORGAN
How long do they think she'll be on the vent?

MS. JENKINS
I doubt she'll ever be getting off of it.

(Silence.)

MORGAN
Has anyone heard from her son Bryce? We sent a telegram to the address she gave me before she went out.

MS. JENKINS
Janet mentioned she'd spoken to him and he should be here in the next week or so. *(Pause.)* Morgan, this is the best place for her. You know and I know the hospital is not the safest place for someone in her condition…the incidence of hospital-acquired infections can be very high, and these patients are so very fragile. Trust me, it's for the best. *(Pause.)* Are we good?

(MORGAN nods. Lights fade to black.)

60

ACT II
SCENE II

(Evening. Two weeks later. Lights up on MORGAN and BRYCE, 40s, standing at the door to AGNES'S room. BRYCE moves to open the door.)

MORGAN

Hold on a second...before you walk through that door you need to be prepared. The last time you saw your mother she was walking and talking; she was eating and drinking on her own. She was independent. You've got to understand that she can't do any of those things now.

(BRYCE leans against the wall for support.)

BRYCE
(Emotionally fatigued--like a sigh.) Shit...

(He slides down the wall and crouches near the floor.)

Oh my god, oh my god, oh my god...

MORGAN

Bryce, let me get you some water, or...there's some coffee in the pantry. Here, why don't you sit down at the desk...

(BRYCE wearily shakes his head. MORGAN exits and returns with a cup of coffee.)

Here...it's a little stale but it does the job. It's ok, have some.

(MORGAN hands the coffee to Bryce.)

Be careful, it's hot. You want sugar?

> *(BRYCE takes the coffee and drinks*
> *quickly from the steaming hot cup; he*
> *burns himself.)*

                    BRYCE
Shit.

                    MORGAN
Are you ok?

> *(BRYCE nods his head.)*

Let me get you some ice.

> *(BRYCE shakes his head no.)*

                    BRYCE
You were sayin' she can't walk...

                    MORGAN
No, she can't walk.

                    BRYCE
She can't speak?

                    MORGAN
No, she can't.

                    BRYCE
She don't eat?

                    MORGAN
Not by herself; there's a tube that goes into her stomach,
and that tube is connected to a bag of nutritional fluid

above her bed. She gets everything she needs through that tube.

BRYCE

Why can't she eat?

MORGAN

She can't eat because she has a different tube in her throat, and that tube is connected to a machine that breathes for her.

BRYCE

I don't get it.

MORGAN

What don't you understand?

BRYCE

(BRYCE pulls himself up to standing.)

Why's she--why's she got some machine breathin' for her?

MORGAN

Your mother is a very sick woman Bryce.

BRYCE

How long's she been like that?

MORGAN

She developed a respiratory infection a little over a month ago. We did the best we could, but her breathing weakened and she had to be sent to the hospital. For a while she seemed to be improving, but then she took a turn for the worse.

                            BRYCE
For the worse…

                            MORGAN
She went into respiratory arrest--that's when she--that's
when she stopped breathing on her own.

                            BRYCE
I want to see her. I want to see her, I want to see--

                            MORGAN
You will Bryce. Please, just give me a minute. You need
to know what to expect.

                            BRYCE
If she come back from the hospital she must have--she
must have healed, right?

                            MORGAN
No, unfortunately she hasn't healed. Bryce, listen,
there's more, and Bryce--some of this--some of this will
shock you. You see, she was in the ICU for over two
weeks, and that--that changes a person. Her face and
body are puffy, and her hands…she's got these special
mittens on her hands…and the mittens…they're attached
to her bedrails…by a strap.

                            BRYCE
By a what?

                            MORGAN
By a strap. She has to be restrained so she won't pull out
any of her tubes.

                    (BRYCE loses his balance a bit.)

Are you ok?

                            64

                    BRYCE
Yeah, I just--I need to--

                    MORGAN
You need to sit.

                    BRYCE
No. I'm ok. I'm ok.

                    MORGAN
I'm so sorry Bryce.

                    BRYCE
How long's she gonna be like that? How long's she
gonna be strapped down like that?

                    MORGAN
It's just a precaution...she'll need it as long as she's on
the ventilator.

                    BRYCE
When's she getting off it?

                    MORGAN
That's not easy for me to answer.

                    BRYCE
Why?

                    MORGAN
When she was hospitalized they treated the underlying
cause--the infection, but there are things we can't
change--things that make it difficult for her to get off the
ventilator.

                    BRYCE
What kind of things?

65

MORGAN

Bryce, your mother smoked for over 50 years, and when
someone smokes the way she did--well, there are long-
term changes that take place in the lungs, there's damage
that can't be reversed.

BRYCE

So what's the plan?

MORGAN

What do you mean?

BRYCE

How we gettin' her back?

MORGAN

Getting her back?

BRYCE

Yeah, so she's walkin' and talkin' again.

MORGAN

Bryce, I don't think you understand…

BRYCE

What don't I understand? I'm askin' when's she gonna
be able to do all those things you were sayin' she can't
do…walkin', talkin', eatin', drinkin'.

MORGAN

You haven't heard a word I've said.

BRYCE

I heard, and I'm sayin' she's in this place payin' good
money and they send her back from the hospital and I
want to know when she's gonna be fixed up.

(MORGAN is silent.)

What's goin' on here?

MORGAN

We're caring for her the best we can, but we can't work miracles. Bryce, there are some important things we need to discuss...before she declines further we need to-

BRYCE

Whoa, what are you sayin'?

MORGAN

I know it's a lot to absorb right now, but--like I said, your mother is a very sick woman.

BRYCE

If she's sick and she's in there on that thing then she just needs to be fixed up, right?

MORGAN

You're a little confused.

BRYCE

I'm not the one who's confused.

MORGAN

Where were you when she was getting sick?

BRYCE

Who the hell do you think you are? I'd have been here if someone woulda told me sooner.

MORGAN

Did you want to be contacted?

BRYCE

You're sayin' I don't care about my Mama?

MORGAN

No, I'm not saying that--

BRYCE

Then what are you sayin' lady?

MORGAN

(Gently.) Bryce, your mother has been my patient for
three months, and in that time I've seen her decline
significantly. It's time for us to sit down and make some
decisions.

BRYCE

I make the decisions.

MORGAN

You're getting in the way.

BRYCE

Huh?!

MORGAN

You can't ignore what's going on here.

BRYCE

(Escalating.) Who the hell do you think you are to be
talking to me like--

MORGAN

Stop. You've been drinking. You need to calm down.

BRYCE

I have not been drinking.

MORGAN

I smell it all over you.

BRYCE

How the hell m' I supposed to be here without drinkin'?

MORGAN

Your mother told me she'd never want to be--that she'd
never want to be dependent on anyone--not like this.

BRYCE

What are you gettin' at?

MORGAN

We need to work together to make sure her wishes are
respected.

BRYCE

You're sayin' she wants us to kill her.

MORGAN

No, that's not what I'm saying.

BRYCE

It's a good thing I came back when I did--what, she's too
expensive? You gonna cut her off?

MORGAN

This isn't a financial issue. It's about the quality of her
life; it's about relieving her suffering; it's about allowing
your mother to have some dignity.

BRYCE

What?

MORGAN

If your mother continues to decline, we need to let her
go comfortably...without a fight.

BRYCE

No. Someone's gotta be fightin' for her.

69

MORGAN

What do you think I'm doing right now?

BRYCE

You want to kill her.

MORGAN

No, it's not like that. *(MORGAN listens to the sound of the ventilators.)* Listen to them--can you hear them?

BRYCE

Hear what?

MORGAN

The ventilators...not just hers, but every patient on this floor. They're a part of them. You can't hear them? The sound pounds away in my head; I hear them in my sleep. The whole floor sounds like some kind of...and we're in the middle of it all--you holding on and me patching them up...everyone here...we're all responsible for making them suffer. Bryce, can't you see--

BRYCE

See what?

MORGAN

There's no hope! Can't you see there's no hope?

(BRYCE exits violently. MORGAN is left alone. Lights fade to black.)

ACT II
SCENE III

(The next day. MS. JENKINS'S office.
MS. JENKINS sits at her desk.
MORGAN enters purposefully.)

MORGAN
You wanted to see me Ms--

MS. JENKINS
What did you say to that woman's son?

MORGAN
What do you mean?

MS. JENKINS
Agnes Jones. Her son stormed into my office this
morning and demanded she be removed from this
facility. He told me you said we were going to stop
caring for his mother.

MORGAN
That's not what I said.

MS. JENKINS
Then what did you say?

MORGAN
I was trying to prepare him. I was only trying to get him
to understand--

MS. JENKINS
You told him he was wrong for--

MORGAN
He's been out of her life for years. His reaction is based
on guilt.

MS. JENKINS
If he feels guilty and we don't act he becomes a liability.

MORGAN
I know what Agnes would have wanted.

MS. JENKINS
Now you're the one making decisions for her?

MORGAN
That's not what I meant; just because we have the technology to keep people alive doesn't mean it's the right way to practice.

MS. JENKINS
That's not what I said. I asked if you were eligible to make decisions for her.

MORGAN
Agnes is a sick woman.

MS. JENKINS
I realize that.

(Phone rings. MS. JENKINS answers.)

No, no. Tell them I'll--tell them I'll get back to them in five minutes.

(MS. JENKINS hangs up the phone.)

MORGAN
We can't keep behaving like she's a healthy woman.

MS. JENKINS
Are you talking about what she wants or what you want? Because it's not about what you want, and I'm not in the business of euthanasia.

MORGAN

I'm not talking about euthanasia; I'm talking about her
rights; she never wanted any of this.

MS. JENKINS

And you know this--how?

MORGAN

She told me.

MS. JENKINS

When?

MORGAN

Before she was sent out she told me she'd never want to
be--

MS. JENKINS

Did she put it on paper?

MORGAN

No.

MS. JENKINS

And why not?

MORGAN

There wasn't time.

MS. JENKINS

Listen to me Ms. Fenster; in case you haven't noticed, I
don't have a crystal ball, and I'm the last person who's
willing to go against the wishes of the family.

MORGAN

Her son has no idea--

MS. JENKINS

If he wants to continue the fight--

MORGAN

It's futile.

MS. JENKINS

It's up to him. *(Pause, she takes a deep breath followed by a forceful exhalation.)*

> *(MS. JENKINS gets up from behind her desk and moves toward MORGAN.)*

I've been a little harsh. I'm sure you can understand, these people, they get upset and then they bring their fury down here to me. *(Pause.)* Let's take a step back. Let me get you--you're a coffee drinker, right? I don't want to take up too much of your time.

> *(MS. JENKINS pours coffee from a carafe. MORGAN waves it away.)*

MORGAN

She's getting worse. That's what I tried to explain to her son.

MS. JENKINS

These situations require a light touch; we don't want to cause the family undue pain. *(Pause.)* I hear you've been talking to a number of our families lately.

MORGAN

I thought that was part of my job.

MS. JENKINS

Mt. Sutton has been caring for the elderly for thirty years. I've been at the helm for the last ten. You've been here for...

74

MORGAN

Three months.

MS. JENKINS

(In a pleasant, mildly sarcastic manner.) Three months
and now you know more than everyone. *(Sweetly.)*
You're making everyone uncomfortable dear. I'm sure
you don't mean to, but we do have a certain way of
doing things around here.

MORGAN

I'm only trying to--

MS. JENKINS

You enjoy working here?

MORGAN

I do. I like the people. *(Clarifying.)* I like the patients.

MS. JENKINS

The patients are why we're here, and we have so many
types of patients in this facility, at all levels of health.
Can you believe Jenny Lee up on three turns one
hundred and seven next week?

MORGAN

What did you say to Agnes's son?

(Pause.)

MS. JENKINS

I told him that she has a strong heart, and that I would do
everything in my power to assure that she lives a long
life.

MORGAN

But that's not right.

75

MS. JENKINS
Medical miracles happen every day.

OVERHEAD
Morgan Fenster, please report to the 8th floor. Morgan
Fenster, please report to the 8th floor.

MORGAN
I need to get back upstairs--

MS. JENKINS
They'll be all right for a moment. *(To the point.)* You're
a bright woman and we all like having you on board, but
there are some things we need to agree on.

MORGAN
What things?

MS. JENKINS
Sometimes the sickest patients require the highest hopes.

MORGAN
What are you saying?

MS. JENKINS
When it comes to life, I believe in the fight. Where
there's struggle, there's life...and there are certain areas
where we must give and we must take.

MORGAN
Give and take?

MS. JENKINS
We need Agnes. We need all of our patients up on eight,
and if we don't keep those beds filled we're going to
have to let some of our people go.

MORGAN

What?

MS. JENKINS

No one who's absolutely essential--one or two of the
recreation staff.

MORGAN

What? If you take any of them away the residents will be
lined up in the hallway staring at the wallpaper.

MS. JENKINS

I'm afraid we'll have no other choice. You've brought it
to my attention that there's not enough nursing staff on
the lower acuity units. Look, how about you leave the
advance directive discussions to us and we'll see what
we can do.

MORGAN

I can't believe I'm hearing this--

MS. JENKINS

This way is better for everyone. You stop talking to the
families and I'll--

MORGAN

I can't do that--

MS. JENKINS

And we'll add some extra staff to help out on the low
acuity floors. I'll even throw in another activities person,
part-time.

MORGAN

And you'll continue adding more vent beds.

MS. JENKINS

If we want extra staff for the patients--

77

MORGAN

This isn't--no! I'm not going to stop talking to the
families, and I am going to do everything I can to--

MS. JENKINS

Ms. Fenster, you are on thin ice. I'm not going to let you
risk our reputation. You work for this company, you
work for me, and you are not going to drag us down with
you.

(Phone rings. MS. JENKINS answers.)

I said I'll be out! *(Pause.)* Oh. *(To MORGAN.)* It's for
you.

(MORGAN takes the phone.)

MORGAN

(Pause.) It's about time. Ok, I'll check my list and see
where we can start. *(Pause.)* What? No, that's
unacceptable--you tell him that! No, tell him we've been
waiting for over two weeks and no one told me he was
coming. *(Silence.)* Ok. All right…we'll do
Agnes…Agnes Jones in 822. Ok, please…can you get
me a couple of number ten blades, some gauze, gloves,
and some drapes? Right. Have them ready.

(She hands the phone to MS. JENKINS.)

The surgeon from Clarkson just showed up…I have to
go. *(Simply.)* They need me.

*(MORGAN exits. MS. JENKINS is left
alone on stage. Lights fade to black.)*

ACT II
SCENE IV

(Lights up on MORGAN and a Licensed
Practical Nurse, 30s.)

MORGAN
I have medication ordered every four hours; there's no
reason for her not to already be--

LPN
PRN.

MORGAN
What?

LPN
PRN. As needed.

MORGAN
Let me see her medication sheet.

> *(The LPN exits. Lights up on AGNES'S*
> *hospital bed. Ventilator is in place and*
> *cranking away. IVs and various items*
> *hang on IV poles. MORGAN stands*
> *beside AGNES'S bedside and observes*
> *her condition. The LPN enters with the*
> *medication card. MORGAN looks it*
> *over.)*

Tylenol?

LPN
Extra strength.

MORGAN
That's all she's had.

79

                    LPN

Ain't that what it says?

                   MORGAN

What about her Percocet? Don't you check to see if she
needs her Percocet?

                    LPN

She can't talk. How'm I supposed to be checkin'?

                   MORGAN

Ok, just…crush the Percocet and give it through her peg
tube.

                         *(The LPN exits. MORGAN tries to rouse
                         AGNES.)*

Agnes?

                   (AGNES stirs.)

Agnes…it's ok, it's ok…we need to look at your wound.

                   (The LPN enters.)

                    LPN

Miss, that surgeon's gonna be down any second.

                   MORGAN

Then he's going to have to wait. Please give her the pain
meds.

                    LPN

Don't think he's gonna--

                   MORGAN

Just do as I say.

(MORGAN goes over to AGNES again.)

It's ok Agnes.

(Using a large syringe, the LPN attempts to put the medication through AGNES'S peg tube but it squirts back at her.)

LPN

Damn. Now I'm gonna have to do it all over again.

(The LPN exits. A SURGEON, 30s, enters.)

MORGAN

We're just giving her some pain meds. She'll need about 30 minutes.

SURGEON

I have to be back by--

MORGAN

There are a couple of other patients upstairs we need to check on. They're not as bad as her, but it'll give us some time for--

SURGEON

I have to be back by eleven. *(Pause.)* What do you want to do?

MORGAN

Can you come back tomorrow?

SURGEON

No.

81

MORGAN

Then when?

SURGEON

I don't know--next week?

MORGAN

They were supposed to send someone a couple of weeks ago. Now she's spiking fevers. We can't wait. No one told us you were coming.

SURGEON

You can send her back up to us and we'll--

MORGAN

Just 20 minutes--

(The SURGEON'S pager goes off. He checks it.)

SURGEON

I can stick around another ten. I need to make a call. Let me know what you want to do.

(The SURGEON exits. MORGAN stares at AGNES. Pause. She puts her hands on the equipment that sits atop the bedside tray table. The LPN enters. MORGAN'S movements take on an automated quality.)

LPN

What you doin' Miss?

MORGAN

We have to get her prepped. Take her ties off--only on the right side…be careful she doesn't pull anything.

82

(They remove half of AGNES'S
restraints. The LPN helps MORGAN
turn AGNES onto her side. They use
pillows to hold her in place. The
SURGEON enters.)

SURGEON

I'm sorry.

MORGAN

No problem.

SURGEON

You have a number fifteen?

MORGAN

We only have tens.

SURGEON

That's fine. Lidocaine?

MORGAN

No.

SURGEON

Nothing to numb--

MORGAN

No.

(The SURGEON removes the dressing.)

SURGEON

(As a sigh.) Ok. *(Pause.)* Where's the trash?

(The LPN grabs the trashcan. The
SURGEON removes AGNES'S soiled
dressing and throws it in the trash. He

examines the wound.)

I need more gauze, a basin, and some irrigation. We really need to clean this out.

(MORGAN holds AGNES on her side as the LPN readies the supplies. MORGAN motions to the LPN.)

MORGAN

Come over here. Hold her--here--no, no--her hands--hold her hands.

(AGNES struggles--at first with quick, sharp movements, and then feebly. They hold her, tightening their grip. The SURGEON picks up the scalpel and looks to MORGAN for approval; MORGAN nods her head and then looks away. The SURGEON'S movements are quick and precise. AGNES'S body jerks sharply and then goes as limp as a rag doll.)

SURGEON

I need that trashcan again.

(MORGAN fortifies her grip on AGNES and motions to the LPN to get the trashcan. The LPN grabs the trashcan and offers it to the SURGEON.)

Irrigation.

(The LPN grabs the irrigating syringe, fills it with saline, and hands it to the SURGEON. He irrigates the wound.)

84

Gauze?

> *(The LPN hands the SURGEON the gauze. She begins to tear off pieces of tape.)*

Thanks.

> *(The SURGEON finishes the procedure and gives MORGAN the ok to return AGNES to her original position.)*

Get her on her side a little.

> *(The LPN props AGNES up on a pillow and leaves the room. The SURGEON removes his gloves and turns to MORGAN.)*

You're the only one here?

> *(MORGAN nods her head.)*

God bless you.

> *(The SURGEON exits. MORGAN stands transfixed. The ventilator alarm goes off. MORGAN silences the alarm. She adjusts AGNES'S position a bit but fails to secure AGNES'S arm restraint. MORGAN turns and sits on a small stool nearby and holds her head in her hands. The alarm on the ventilator goes off again. AGNES has pulled the tube out of her throat and now holds it in her hand. MORGAN jumps up, grabs hold of AGNES'S arm, and pries the breathing tube out of AGNES'S hand.)*

85

With difficulty, she forces AGNES'S arm onto the bedrail and secures the restraint. MORGAN moves to replace the breathing tube when she locks eyes with AGNES. AGNES grunts and moves her head from side to side to indicate 'no'. MORGAN nods, whispers into AGNES'S ear, smooths her hair, and stares into AGNES'S eyes while continuing to hold the breathing tube in her hand. The sound of the alarm continues as lights fade to black.)

ACT II
SCENE V

(Five days later. Lights up on a bright white room. MORGAN is seated at a metal table. RALPH HAWKINS, 50s, her defense attorney, sits across from her.)

HAWKINS
You need to stay quiet. Do you understand? I can help you if you do what I say.

MORGAN
You don't realize what's happening out there. The jury has to hear my story. People need to hear what I have to say.

HAWKINS
We discussed that you would take the 5th on all questions posed before your evaluation. You agreed to this.

MORGAN
Yes, I agreed but--

HAWKINS
I speak. You do not.

MORGAN
They're going to write me off. I don't want people to think I'm crazy. They need to understand why I did what I did. What about my story? What about Agnes's story?

HAWKINS
Morgan--

MORGAN
People need to understand--

87

HAWKINS

If this goes to trial--

MORGAN

You've got to help me. No one will know the truth about
what goes on in these places if you don't--

HAWKINS

They are not on trial Morgan. You are.

MORGAN

They answer to no one.

HAWKINS

They are regulated by the state. In 2008, Mt. Sutton was
found to have only five deficiencies.

MORGAN

Only!!!

HAWKINS

In comparison to similar homes, Mt. Sutton ranks within
the top--

MORGAN

That's bullshit. What is the state *doing* about it? What is
the law *doing* about it? The state comes in and we put on
a dog and pony show; disinfect the place with pine
scented air freshener to cover up the smell of human
garbage; prop all the residents up, line em' up in the
hallways--

HAWKINS

Mt. Sutton ranks within the acceptable range of--

MORGAN

Acceptable--what's that supposed to mean? Acceptable
to whom? The place where my grandmother was--they

had deficiencies, "acceptable deficiencies." She was overmedicated…took her wheelchair down a flight of stairs that should have been gated. Oh yeah, the state gave them high marks. We treat dogs better than old people.

HAWKINS
They're saying that you violently extubated that patient and then watched as she suffocated, that you watched and did nothing. They have witnesses who will testify against you. Her son says you wanted his mother dead; the staff says you insisted on a procedure that took place without any anesthetic, and Ms. Francine Jenkins--she describes your behavior as erratic. *(Pause.)* Morgan, did--did your grandmother's death set you off?

MORGAN
My grandmother's death didn't set me off. Her death made me dedicate myself to people just like her.

HAWKINS
Just like--

MORGAN
Innocent, vulnerable. *(Agitated.)* Ventilators, 'terminal life support.' Can't speak because they got a tube here. *(She points to her throat.)* Can't make a sound, it's like you don't exist. I figured it out! Everybody's wrong--the hospitals, the doctors, the families--everybody's wrong! No one listens to *nature*, no one listens to what these patients want--*need*. Those machines are meant to save viable life, to make it better--not to prolong it, not to extend suffering.

HAWKINS
But Morgan--

MORGAN

Nobody wants to know what happens in these homes,
nobody wants to admit there's no end to disease, that
death is not something that can be overcome. Just
because we have the technology doesn't mean we
always need to use it. People don't realize that this could
happen to them.

HAWKINS

Even if I let you testify...once they start calling
witnesses, the image of you holding her breathing tube
will be etched in everyone's mind. If you don't take this
opportunity--Morgan, at trial they are not going to hold
back. They're going to ask you "how did you go from
caring for Agnes to killing her?"

MORGAN

(MORGAN slowly relives the moment.) Agnes came
back from the hospital and she had this terrible bedsore--
all dead, all dead tissue; down to the muscle tissue, down
to the bone. It was so big you could put your fist right
into it. When she was readmitted I went in with the
nurses to do the dressing change; I walked into her room
and they were all gasping for breath and shouting
"Damn, she stinks! Grab the peppermint, grab the
peppermint! Cut the stink in here." Of course Agnes
heard everything. *(Pause.)* Not long after, she started
spiking fevers. The wound was infected and her life was
in danger. We had to cut the infection out of her body.
(Pause.) When the surgeon arrived...I shut down and
I...I felt like a machine. I had her prepped, and I held her
on her side, and I...I was looking into her eyes, and her
eyes were just like my grandmother's eyes; and her eyes
were telling me, and her body was telling me she was
suffering, and the surgeon hesitated but I gave him the
sign to go ahead, and when he did...her mouth opened
and it was all contorted but nothing came out...on
account of the tube. *(Pause.)* Afterwards...I whispered

to her that I would help her, and that she'd never have to feel pain like that again.

(Silence.)

(A GUARD enters.)

Mr. Hawkins, I'm not afraid to die; what I do fear is that none of this will ever stop, that suffering will continue being prolonged, and that more money will be spent on inventing machines than caring for the people who are attached to those machines. Please--you--the law--the state--someone's got to help them. You've got to do something. Do something.

> *(The GUARD escorts MORGAN out of the room. Lights dim. Spotlight on HAWKINS as he turns to face the audience. Lights slowly fade to black.)*

END OF PLAY